Lose Weight by Walking:

An Easy Guide to Better Fitness, Health and Happiness

By

Larry S. Hiller

Table of contents

Introduction

Walking is one of the most well-known types of activity around the world. It doesn't need costly hardware or extraordinary abilities, and it gives an extensive variety of medical advantages. Whether you pick an open air route in nature, a bustling course on city walkways, a treadmill exercise, or a couple of rounds around your place of business, walking is a moderately available method for remaining dynamic.

Walking is a kind of cardiovascular physical activity which expands your pulse. This further develops the blood stream and can bring down circulatory strain. It assists with supporting energy levels by delivering specific chemicals like endorphins and conveying oxygen all through the body. Energetic walking is viewed as a moderate-force, low-influence exercise that doesn't apply overabundant burden on joints (hip, knee, lower legs) that are defenseless to injury with higher-influence exercises.

Individuals might imagine that walking isn't generally as compelling as higher-influence exercises. However an enormous companion investigation of sprinters and walkers tracked down that following 6 years of follow-up, while exhausting an equivalent measure of energy, moderate-power offered comparative advantages as higher-force running in diminishing the gamble of hypertension, elevated cholesterol, and diabetes. The quicker the walking pace, the more noteworthy the gamble decrease noticed.

Walking and Well-being

The 2018 Physical Activity Rules for Americans suggests that grown-ups with persistent circumstances do somewhere around 150-300 minutes of moderate-power oxygen consuming exercises week after week, if capable. Walking is an activity that meets this oxygen consuming part and is related with further developing hypertension and weight record, and bringing down the gamble of diabetes, stroke, and cardiovascular infection, and early passing. Walking velocity, length, and recurrence can be changed relying upon one's beginning wellness level, so that nearly everybody can take part in walking as exercise.

Is achieving 10000 steps a day compulsory?

You've most likely heard that moving 10,000 steps a day is a solid objective. Some applications and pedometers have 10,000 steps reserved, so that when you arrive at it, a congratulatory message is seen. Not a straightforward objective as a considerable lot of us sit more than stand, because of driving vehicles, sitting at office work areas, and leaning back in seats at home; as a matter of fact the normal number of day to day steps an American takes is more like 4,800. It might shock you that the benchmark number of 10,000 isn't really founded on science however was made as a showcasing strategy during the 1960s by an organization making pedometers.

So is there any science to help venturing it up? For the most part, research observes that more advances are better however even a lower sum can accomplish medical advantages. A review following 4,840 people 40 years old and more established for around 10 years found that those making something like 8,000 steps day to day had a 51% lower passing rate from all causes contrasted than those making 4,000 steps or less. An excess of 16,000 more established American ladies from the Ladies' Wellbeing Study followed for a considerable length of time found that those requiring 4,400 steps a day had a 41% lower passing rate contrasted than those making around 2,700 steps every day. Passing rates kept on dropping corresponding to making more steps up to 7,500 day to day, however ventures past that didn't show extra advantage.

Albeit these investigations affirm that making more steps is great, they specifically add up to see a medical advantage that will fluctuate among people. The rule from the Communities for Infectious prevention and Counteraction to "move more and sit less over the course of the day; some exercise is superior to none" stays a suitable objective for everybody. Nothing bad can really be said about holding back nothing or significantly higher, with the exception of when it turns out to be overwhelming to such an extent that you lose inspiration or you feel deterred that a lesser sum isn't sufficient. As opposed to feeling fastened to a particular step count, pay attention to your body, challenge it, and be happy-go-lucky about what it can achieve.

Chapter 1

Hazards of an inactive lifestyle

An idle way of life can be described in different ways such as being a habitual slouch, not working out, being in a stationary state most of the time. You have most likely known about these expressions, and they mean exactly the same thing: a way of life with a ton of sitting and resting, with very little to no activity.

In the US and all over the planet, individuals are investing increasingly more energy doing stationary exercises. During our recreation time, we are in many cases sitting: while at the same time utilizing a PC or other gadget, staring at the television, or playing computer games. A considerable lot of our positions have become more stationary, with long days sitting at a work area. Furthermore, the way the vast majority of us get around includes sitting - in vehicles, on transports, and on trains.

Driving a stationary way of life is turning into a huge general medical problem. Stationary ways of life seem, by all accounts, to be progressively far and wide in numerous countries notwithstanding being connected to a scope of ongoing medical issue.

A great many people carrying on with a stationary way of life are probably not going to meet the public exercise standards. As per the public authority's 2008 Exercise Rules for Americans, grown-ups ought to get no less than 150 minutes of moderate-power exercise every week.

A 2017 paper by the Stationary Conduct Exploration Organization (SBRN) characterized inactive way of behaving as any action including sitting, leaning back, or resting that has extremely low energy consumption. The estimation for energy consumption is metabolic eciprocals (METs), and the creators consider exercises hat exhaust 1.5 METs or less of energy to be stationary.

Research recommends that main 21% of grown-ups are neeting the exercise standards, while fewer than 5% perform 30 minutes of exercise each day.

Risks of a stationary way of life

A stationary way of life can add to stoutness, diabetes, and a few kinds of disease.

Late exploration is beginning to affirm the wellbeing gambles related with an inactive way of life.

Studies have now reliably shown the way that driving a stationary way of life can add to:

Corpulence

Type 2 diabetes

Cardiovascular illness

Untimely passing

Broadened times of inertia can lessen metabolism and hinder the body's capacity to control glucose levels, direct pulse, and stall fat.

A review dissected information gathered for 15 years and observed that inactive ways of life were related with an expanded gamble of early passing due to paying little heed to exercise.

This shows that it is fundamental to lessen how much time spent being stationary as well as doing more activity.

Emotional wellness

A stationary way of life likewise seems to adversely affect mental prosperity. The mix of the physical and mental effect on wellbeing makes an inactive way of life especially risky. A review with 10,381 members related an inactive way of life and absence of exercise with a higher gamble of fostering a psychological well-being problem. A new survey that included information from 110,152 members tracked down a connection between stationary way of behaving and an expanded gamble of despondency. Actual idleness, along expanding tobacco use and less than stellar eating routine and nourishment, are progressively turning out to be essential for the present way of life prompting the fast ascent of sicknesses like cardiovascular illnesses, diabetes, or weight. Persistent sicknesses brought about by these gamble factors are currently the main sources of death in all aspects of world with the exception of sub-Saharan Africa, where irresistible illnesses, for example, Helps are as yet the main issue. These ongoing illnesses are, generally, actually preventable.

Dangers of an inactive way of life

Vein-related issue: When you don't move enough, your blood stream eases back, this might possibly bring about blood clumps. Being actually dynamic can assist you with staying away from blood clumps hindering the veins close to your essential organs, like your heart.

Coronary illness, elevated cholesterol and hypertension: When a person is in a stationary state for a long time, it's conceivable that unsaturated fats might develop in veins, which might influence heart wellbeing and raise cholesterol and pulse. It's suggested that grown-ups and youngsters do something like 2.5 long stretches of exercise each week to diminish the opportunity for these issues to happen. In any case, ongoing examinations have shown that only one out of five grown-ups and teenagers get the suggested measure of activity.

Particular kinds of malignant growth: Stationary way of behaving may expand the gamble of creating endometrial, ovarian and different tumors. Turning out to be more dynamic and, surprisingly, possibly changing your eating routine might assist you with decreasing disease gambles.

Psychological dangers: Stress, uneasiness and melancholy when truly dynamic, your cerebrum discharges serotonin, which is a temperament supporting compound in your mind. Without exercise, less serotonin is delivered, so you might have less good sentiments and less inspiration. At the point when you have less inspiration, dealing with your psychological wellness might turn out to be more troublesome. While this can be a moving cycle to explore, there are steps you can take to work on your emotional well-being and prosperity.

Chapter 2

Walking and its Advantages

Walking is an extraordinary method for improving or keeping up with your general wellbeing. Only 30 minutes consistently can increment cardiovascular wellness, reinforce bones, decrease overabundant muscle fat, and lift muscle power and perseverance. It can likewise lessen your gamble of creating conditions like coronary illness, type 2 diabetes, osteoporosis and tumors. Unlike a few different types of activities, walking is free and requires no unique gear or preparing.

Exercise doesn't need to be overwhelming or accomplished for extensive stretches to work on your wellbeing. A 2007 investigation of latent ladies tracked down that even a low degree of activity - around 75 minutes out of every week - further developed their wellness levels essentially, when contrasted with a non-practicing bunch.

Walking is low effect, requires negligible gear, should be possible whenever of day and can be performed at your own speed. You can get out and walk without agonizing over the dangers related for certain more fiery types of activity. Walking is likewise an extraordinary type of exercise for individuals who are overweight, older, or who haven't practiced in quite a while.

Walking for the sake of entertainment and wellness isn't restricted to walking around nearby neighborhood roads. There are different clubs, scenes and methodologies you can use to make walking an agreeable and social piece of your way of life.

Benefits of Walking

- Forestall or oversee different circumstances, including coronary illness, stroke, hypertension, malignant growth and type 2 diabetes
- Work on cardiovascular wellness
- Fortify your bones and muscles
- Further develop muscle perseverance
- Increment energy levels
- Work on your mind-set, perception, memory and rest
- Work on your equilibrium and coordination
- Reinforce invulnerable framework
- Lessen pressure and strain

The quicker, farther and all the more as often as possible you walk, the more prominent the advantages. For instance, you might begin as a normal walker, and afterward move gradually up to walking quicker and walking a mile in a more limited measure of time than a typical walker, like power walkers. This can be an extraordinary method for getting oxygen consuming action, further develop your heart wellbeing and increment your perseverance while consuming calories.

You can likewise substitute times of energetic walking with relaxed walking. This kind of stretch preparation has many advantages, like working on cardiovascular wellness and consuming a bigger number of calories than standard walking. Also, span preparing should be possible quicker than ordinary walking

Walking can offer various medical advantages to individuals of any age and wellness levels. It might likewise assist with forestalling specific illnesses and even draw out your life. Walking is something that should be treated as a daily practice. All you really need to commence walking is a durable sets of walking shoes.

Peruse on to find out about a portion of the advantages of walking.

1. Burning calories

Walking can assist you with consuming calories. Consuming calories can help you keep up with or get in shape. Your real calorie shedding will rely upon a few elements, including: Walking speed, distance covered, landscape (you'll burn a greater number of calories walking uphill than you'll burn on a level surface due to the extra effort it takes to move uphill).

2. Reinforce the heart

Walking no less than 30 minutes a day, five days a week, can diminish your gamble for coronary illness by around 19 percent. Furthermore, your chances of coronary heart diseases reduce significantly more when you increment the length or distance you walk each day.

3. Can assist with bringing down your blood sugar

Going for a short walk subsequent to eating might assist with bringing down your blood sugar. A little report found that going for a 15-minute walk three times each day (after breakfast, lunch, and supper) further developed blood sugar levels more than going for a 45-minute walk at one more point during the day. Consider making a post-feast walk a normal piece of your daily schedule. It can likewise assist you with fitting practice in over the course of the day.

4. Facilitates joint agony

Walking can assist with safeguarding the joints, including your knees and hips. That is on the grounds that it greases up and fortifies the muscles that help the joints. Walking may likewise give advantages to individuals living with joint inflammation, like decreasing agony. What's more, Walking 5 to 6 miles a week may likewise assist with forestalling joint pain.

5. Helps respiratory organs

Walking may decrease your chances of catching a cold or influenza. One review followed 1,000 grown-ups during influenza season. The individuals who walked at a moderate speed for 30 to 45 minutes daily had 43% less days off and less upper respiratory lot contaminations by and large. Their side effects were likewise decreased assuming they became ill. That was contrasted with grown-ups in the review who were stationary.

Attempt a day to day walk to encounter these advantages. In the event that you live in a cool environment, you can attempt to walk on a treadmill or move around an indoor shopping center.

6. Helps in boosting morale

No mystery practice is a well-informed and demonstrated method for decreasing pressure. Walking discharges endorphins, a vibe decent compound in the body that advances a condition of delight like chuckling and love. "Endorphins collaborate with receptors in the mind and achieve sensations of prosperity, expanded confidence, expanded torment resilience, and, surprisingly, a feeling of elation, frequently alluded to as a 'sprinter's high,'" Dr. Lam makes sense of.

Walking genuinely encourages you. A recent report found that even single, brief 10-minute episodes of walking further developed the mind-set condition of members.

To begin Walking, all you'll require is a couple of durable walking shoes. Pick a mobile course close to your home. Or on the other hand search for a grand spot to walk like a path or on the ocean front.

You can likewise enroll a companion or relative to walk with you. On the other hand, you can add walking into your everyday daily schedule. Here are a few thoughts:

Assuming you drive, get off your transport or train one stop early and walk the remainder of the distance. Leave farther away from your office than expected and walk to and from your vehicle. Consider walking as opposed to driving when you get things done. You can follow through with your jobs and fit in practice simultaneously. Walking can satisfy day to day suggested practices for individuals of any age and wellness levels. Consider getting a pedometer or other wellness tracker to monitor your day to day advances. Pick a mobile course and day to day step objective that is proper for your age and wellness level. Warm up prior to walking to prevent joint stiffness and any other complication that comes with walking. Continuously address your PCP prior to beginning another wellness schedule.

Chapter 3

Maintaining a proper walking/work out habit

We as a whole realize an everyday walking propensity is certainly worth staying aware of for its physical and psychological well-being benefits. You've most likely heard the counsel to plan your walks in your schedule or set out your shoes the prior night. Perhaps you've even taken a stab at dozing in your walking outfit, so you have no real reason to skirt your morning walk. Yet, in some cases, notwithstanding our best goals, getting out the entryway for a walk can feel close to unimaginable.

To increment inspiration when you're not feeling it, take a stab at moving your mentality with these methods:

1. Adhere to THE 10-MINUTE Guideline

Make a deal with yourself. "Let yourself know you simply need to walk for 10 minutes," recommends Amy Morin, a psychotherapist and host of the Intellectually Resilient Individuals digital recording. "If you would rather not continue onward, you can stop. More often than not, you'll decide to continue onward. Beginning is generally the hardest part."

2. MAKE Walking YOUR Prize

Rather than considering walking something you need to do, shift your language and consider it a prize. "Rather than 'I ought to get out for a walk,' attempt 'I get to take a walk,'" suggests Karin Cleary, PhD, an authorized clinician. This functions admirably in the event that you use walking as a method for compensating yourself for a useful block of work. "Plan to work briefly, and afterward you get to have some time off and take a walk." Doing so can consequently assist with supporting your imagination and efficiency at work.

3. Attempt a Smaller than usual Test

"Set a little test for yourself every week, such as walking 5 minutes more than the other day," says Kelly Keck, LMHC, a psychotherapist. You can likewise have a go at adding .25 miles or 1,000 additional moves toward your day. Another incredible choice: "Challenge your companions to see who can make all the more day to day steps since responsibility is an immense inspiration," says Keck. At the point when you start little with feasible successes, you'll feel more engaged to keep on arriving at greater objectives.

4. Enroll an Accomplice

"It very well may be a relative, companion or even your pet," says Ben Reuter, PhD, ensured strength and molding trained professional and exercise physiologist. "This helps consider you responsible and makes it more pleasant. My responsibility accomplices are two Labrador retrievers. Awful climate, when I'm probably going to rationalize, is the point at which they flourish with walks."

5. Consolidate YOUR Walk WITH SOMETHING YOU Believe that Should DO

"Something that gets me out the entryway for a long walk, particularly when I'm not in that frame of mind, and I simply need to veg on the lounge chair, is to join it with an action I truly would like to do," says Jonathan Jordan, an ensured fitness coach. "For example, I'll involve it as a chance to chat on the telephone with my closest companion or mother, or I'll make the objective a spot I love." That could be your number one café or book shop, for instance.

6. Rethink YOUR Outlook ABOUT YOUR WALK

Rather than considering your walk an exercise, consider it moving your body. "Advising yourself to move today seems like less strain than advising yourself to take a long walk," makes sense of Susan Masterson, MPH, PhD, an authorized therapist. "Just 'moving is something you can expand on and doesn't have the achievement disappointment meaning to it."

7. Join YOUR Walk TO A Laid out Propensity

In the event that you consistently battle to get out for a walk, it can assist with attaching your walk onto another propensity you don't battle with. "On the off chance that you're doing likewise consistently, such as having breakfast, take a stab at walking before or after," recommends Leeann Rybakov, a wellbeing mentor. "Simply matching it with something you as of now will make it almost certain that the propensity will stick."

8. KEEP A Rundown OF REASONS YOU Believe that Should WALK

Being helped to remember your "why" for walking can make it more straightforward to get up and out. "Make a rundown of the relative multitude of motivations behind why walking is really great for you — like it's great for your heart, and it gives you energy," says Morin. "Whenever you're enticed to skirt your walk, read the rundown. It'll assist you with moving back that multitude of reasons, and give you the inspiration you want to make it happen."

9. Investigate Another Course

On the off chance that fatigue's the issue, stir up your walking areas. "Attempt another spot each time you take a walk" recommends Bianca Grover, an activity physiologist. "Walking a similar path could get old for a few of us. Track down another park or another neighborhood to keep things fascinating". The progression in territory (like slopes) additionally helps to work different muscle gatherings.

10. At any rate, review a Period YOU WEREN'T Spurred, Yet Walked

Remind yourself what happened the last time you felt like this, however chose to feel free to go for your walk, suggests Evan Lawrence, an ensured fitness coach. "How could you feel a while later? You felt perfect eventually!

Furthermore, you were so happy you got it done. You did it previously, and you can rehash it."

11. Make IT Stride BY-STEP

Now and again, we take on such a large number of new wellbeing propensities on the double, leaving us feeling paralyzed by all the change. Assuming walking is your fundamental need, center just around that. "Tell yourself, all I'm doing is adding a walk. I don't need to transform anything more,'" says Elisabeth Goldberg, an

authorized marriage and family specialist. "Change can be exceptionally overwhelming and can put activity down. It doesn't need to be win big or bust, particularly while you're expecting to roll out long haul improvements."

12. Indulge YOURSELF

It could sound senseless; however having a prize sitting tight for you toward the finish of your walk really exploits a criticism circle incorporated into our minds. The prize doesn't need to be anything huge. "For instance I, in the same way as other others, partake in my morning mug espresso," says Andrew Swasey, a confirmed fitness coach. "So I utilize a prompt, everyday practice, reward cycle to compensate myself with some espresso after my walk. My sign is to begin my espresso producer, my routine is to take my walk, and my prize is to drink some espresso in the wake of returning home from my walk." Or on the other hand on the off chance that you like to walk in the nights, perhaps your award is loosening up with a hot shower.

13. TALK As though YOU Realize THE WALK WILL Occur

How you converse with yourself as well as other people about your Walking plans can be the contrast between adhering to them and not. Have a go at making statements like: "After my espresso, I take my walk and afterward prepare for work," or "I'm taking a walk after supper," prompts Jennifer Branstetter, an authorized clinical social specialist. "This is not quite the same as saying, 'I need to take a walk later,' 'I want to take a walk,' or something less concrete. Try not to give your cerebrum the decision, since offered the chance, your mind will work you out of it."

14. FIND an Explanation Greater THAN YOURSELF

Demonstrations of administration can super rouse. "So frequently, we will accomplish for others how might be challenging to help ourselves," brings up Karina Krepp, a fitness coach. "I challenge my clients to find a companion who needs a walk much more than they do. Somebody you realize who just had hip medical procedure? Assist them with their recommended walking treatment. A companion brings in close to home pain? Ribbon up and meet them for a walk around the recreation area." Recently, Krepp has been going through her morning walk carrying food to her nearby local area refrigerator. Whether you log miles for your #1 cause or are assisting a companion or relative, make your walk part of how you offer in return.

You are in good company! There are a large number of other people who need to practice consistently, however find it challenging to remain spurred or intrigued. However physical as exercise may be, the initial step to any sort of activity is your psychological state. It is vital to recollect that you work out, not to torment yourself, but rather to encourage yourself. Customary activity has been related with so many medical advantages, it is astounding that not more individuals practice consistently. Concentrates show that exercise increment your life expectancy, brings down pulse, diminishes the gamble of different malignant growths, and even upgrades your temperament. When you start your work-out daily practice, you will see that your body is more appealing; however you will likewise have more energy to do the things you love.

Chapter 4

Prevalent Walking Worries and their Remedies

A devoted walking system can assist you with shedding pounds, fabricate more grounded muscles, and improve cardio perseverance. Similarly as with an activity, you could experience specific obstructions during preparing.

The following are 10 normal walking issues and straightforward guidance for settling them so you can keep your walking routine on target.

1. Knee Pain

On the off chance that you're encountering knee torment during or after a walk, a decent spot to begin is with your footwear. Having a legitimate walking shoe that ıccommodates your foot accurately and transforming it ɜach 500-600 miles can assist with forestalling knee orment. You'll likewise need to ensure you're not over striding and increment your absolute week by week nileage by something like 10% every week to permit vour body to adjust to the movement.

Ǝxtending post-walk can likewise assist with further leveloping adaptability and icing sensitive areas can lecrease irritation. In the event that the issue continues, t's smart to talk with a clinical expert.

2. Energy loss

n the event that you need more energy to traverse a walk, nvestigate what you're eating (or not) pre-exercise. Decide on straightforward starches that can without much of a stretch be processed before an exercise. "For exercises under 60 minutes, a little tidbit like a banana or piece of toast would get the job done," says Stephanie Nelson, an enrolled dietitian and MyFitnessPal's in-house sustenance master. In the event that you're walking for over an hour or increasing the power, you might require extra fuel like a little piece of cereal or a smoothie. You can try different things with what turns out best for your body by following your food and noticing how you feel.

3. Time is scarce

Regardless of whether you just have 10 minutes, you can in any case get in a decent exercise. One simple method for expanding the amount of calories you burn, get more grounded and make your walks more troublesome is to stir things up around town and exploit slants, which work more muscle gatherings. You can likewise incorporate short, focused energy spans where you hurry up a few times during your walk. One more method for adding more test: Incorporate walking rushes, step-ups on a recreation area seat and other bodyweight works out.

4. Downplaying the ability of walking

Walking is frequently misjudged and can be similarly comparable to running for heart wellbeing. It's likewise simpler on the joints and more available for individuals of any age and capacities. To up your walking power, go for the gold speed or around 100 steps each moment.

5. Pushing the limit too much

Albeit more uncertain than other high-intensity games like running or cycling, expanding your walking mileage excessively fast can make you over train and lead to injury. Essentially, including an excessive number of spans or speeding up excessively fast without sufficient recuperation time between exercises can likewise be tricky. In the event that you're feeling firm or sore prior to going out on a walk, this might be a sign you want more rest between exercises.

6. Side stitches/fastens

Side fastens are brought about by a fit of the stomach. This can occur during quick breathing, so, on the off chance that a side line becomes excruciating, decline your speed or quit walking to let your breathing get back to business as usual. Expanding your speed excessively fast while starting your walk can cause side lines, so heating up to a quicker pace progressively could assist with forestalling this. Eating and drinking a great deal before your exercise can likewise cause side fastens, so try different things with how much liquid and food you're polishing off preceding your walk.

7. Boredom

Take a stab at changing everything around with various courses and landscapes; on the off chance that that isn't a choice as a result of time imperatives, have a go at walking with an accomplice or joining a mobile club. Another choice is to pay attention to music, a book recording or a digital broadcast to keep you occupied intellectually.

8. The Weather Isn't On Your Side

In the mid-year, walking in the early morning or late night might assist you with combatting warm climate. In the event that your body isn't responding great to the temps, have a go at going for more limited walks over the course of the day. Additionally, in the event that it's excessively sweltering or cold out (or there's nasty weather conditions), the treadmill or walking inside are go-to choices also. At-home Walking exercises are additionally useful.

9. Oblivious To the Required Amount of Water to Consume

How much water you want to drink during an exercise is individual and can rely upon factors like how hot and sticky it is that day, the amount you gauge and your own perspiration rate. One way you can decide whether you're drinking sufficient water and the amount you really want to drink a short time later is to gauge yourself when your walk. For each pound of weight you lose, you'll have to drink around 16 ounces of water to recharge what you've lost. A couple of pounds of weight reduction are typical for a really long time or extraordinary exercises, yet in the event that you're losing more than this, you might have to expand your admission during exercise. On the off chance hat you notice a ton of salt buildup all over or body ollowing a walk, you might have to supplant the sodium ou're losing too. For this situation (or for walks longer han 60 minutes), you ought to consider a games drink to ehydrate.

10. Post-Workout Irritations

rritation is ordinary, despite the fact that assuming it eeps you from actually working, you might have to add nore recuperation time. However long your irritation lisappears following a little while, there ought not to be a ot to stress over. Icing post-exercise, extending, and equiring a little while off until your irritation dies down s the suggested guidance generally speaking. On the off hance that your touchiness is solely after lengthy or xtraordinary exercises, a simple, short recuperation walk the next day can assist with jump-starting the system and facilitate a portion of the irritation.

Chapter 5

Walking styles and posture

Did you know that there are different ways to walk? Yes you heard me correctly. Apparently, there isn't an ideal way to walk. There are different styles that serve different purposes and can be used at one's jurisdiction.

Brisk Walking

Walking is an extraordinary cardio practice both inside and outside. Specialists propose going for the gold pulse in light of your age or around 100 steps each moment to get the most medical advantages. One more method for telling you're walking quickly enough: Work without holding back while walking. "At the point when you take an energetic walk, you will begin to feel somewhat short of breath, in spite of the fact that you ought to in any case have the option to hold down a discussion," says Paul Gent of Walking Foundation. It's wise to do a little extending when you set out, so you don't cause yourself any wounds. You need to set off at a speed that is faster than your consistent walk, yet that you can keep up for about 60 minutes.

Nordic Walking

Nordic Walking is like skiing without skis. Walkers utilize two shafts to push down starting from the earliest stage, out additional muscles than a typical walk does. "It is fundamental that your shafts are the right length, and they can be utilized both on hard surfaces like asphalts as well as the more normal fields out in the open country," Gent says. "Nordic Walking is regularly famous among additional older walkers, as they partake in the dependability that the posts offer."

Marathon Walking

However long distance races are past normal in 2021, a portion of these 26-mile courses offer walkers an opportunity to contend at a more slow speed. The 2019 London Long distance race allowed members an opportunity to investigate Britain's capital another way. The course included parks, streams and notorious tourist spots, for example, the Pinnacle of London, Buckingham Castle, the Places of Parliament and the London Eye. "Everyone walks at various rates yet, all things considered, least of 6 hours with 8 being more normal," Gent says. "Obviously, some will take more time, so setting to the side the entire day for your efforts is ideal."

Chi Walking

Chi walking style centers more on integrating Tai Chi developments into your walk. It's a low-effect and agony free method for working on your wellbeing, as indicated by Body Stream. This structure is an incredible option for those restoring from a sickness or injury. It underlines great stance, free joints, drawing in the center, and loosening up the arms and legs, per Body Streams.

Race Walking

Race Walking is a step above power walking, however with some contest blended into the routine. From youth sports to Olympics Games, race Walking is challenged in all degrees of Olympic style events. Racers should keep in touch with the ground consistently, with the main leg ixed as the foot connects with the ground. "Assuming you have seen race walking on the television while watching the Olympics, you will see that their walking stride is exceptionally misrepresented," Gent says. "There's a genuine wobble from one side to another. It generally makes individuals snicker, however it tends to be habit-forming to watch."

Power Walking

A little faster than brisk walking, this walk requires moving your twisted arms to speed up. "It's turning into an option in contrast to running, as individuals understand the impacts of running can have on joints and feet," Gent says. "It has been recommended that power walking burns off however many calories as running, so it is an extraordinary choice to take if attempting to get thinner." Likewise, Rebecca Stanborough of Healthline suggests walkers get the right stuff, find and study the format of a decent walking way, and get a mobile mate to make it more tomfoolery.

Importance of proper walking technique and posture

How you hold your body is a significant consider having the option to walk serenely and without any problem. Having a legitimate walking stance will make it more straightforward to inhale simpler and walk quicker and farther. Assuming you've had issues appreciating walking in light of the fact that you feel a throbbing painfulness subsequently, the principal thing to check is your stance and how you convey your head and shoulders. As a little something extra, further developing your walking stance will make you look longer, sure, and fit. It's a moment overhaul for zero expense — only a bit of training and care. Improving and keeping up with great stance will prove to be useful whether you're Walking outside or on a treadmill at the rec center.

Steps on how to achieve a proper walking posture

Put yourself in a position for the right stance before you start walking. Spending the initial 15 seconds of your walking meeting zeroing in on great stance will give you a vastly improved exercise. Be that as it may, it doesn't end there. Occasionally check in with yourself and ensure you're carrying out the vital steps to accomplish legitimate stance until it turns into a propensity.

Stand upright: Envision being tall and straight, similar to a tree. Try not to slump or curve your back.

Try not to incline forward or back: Resting overburdens the back muscles as you walk, and you ought to abstain from inclining with the exception of when on a slope. While walking uphill, it's okay to incline somewhat forward (never in reverse) from the lower legs. Walking downhill, you can likewise incline somewhat forward or keep a straight back. In the two circumstances, you need to try not to recline or excessively far forward with the goal that you don't tumble off balance.

Keep your eyes forward: Abstain from peering down. Your center ought to be around 20 feet in front of you. Along these lines, you will see your way and anything coming at you from the side.

Keep your head up (lined up with the ground): This lessens burden on your neck and back. A legitimate jawline position will likewise permit you to look forward as opposed to down at your feet.

Loosen your shoulders: Shrug once and permit your shoulders to fall and unwind, somewhat back. Relaxing the shoulders will assist with easing pressure and put them into a situation to utilize great arm movement while walking. You can likewise do this at spans during your walk to guarantee you are keeping your shoulders loose.

Keep a fixed core: Your center muscles can assist you with keeping up with great stance and oppose slumping and inclining. Keeping your stomach pulled in marginally (while as yet taking profound, full breaths) can assist you with keeping a decent walking stance.

Neutral pelvis: You need to ensure your hips are not shifting forward or back while you're walking. Work on staying your butt out, wrapping it up, and afterward seeing as a characteristic center. The center is where you need to be. This will hold you back from curving your back.

By implementing the various walking styles and maintaining a good walking posture, you are sure to lose weight and minimize the various complications that come with walking. Remember to not strain yourself excessively. Take breaks when you need to do so; your body isn't a machine, it requires rest. Make sure to take a break when you feel like you need one.

So far we have been able to cover the **walking aspect** of losing weight. The subsequent chapter will be talking about the **diet aspect** of weight loss.

Chapter 6

Calories and nutrition

Weight control is fundamentally one thing — calories. Indeed, even with all the eating regimen plans out there, weight management actually boils down to the calories you take in versus those you burn off during movement. Famous craze diets might guarantee you that not eating starches (carbs) or eating a heap of grapefruit is the key to weight reduction. Be that as it may, it truly comes down to eating fewer calories than your body is utilizing to get more fit. Calories are the energy in food. Your body has a steady interest for energy and utilizes the calories from food to continue to work. Energy from calories energizes all your activities, from squirming to long distance race running.

Sugars, fats and proteins are the kinds of supplements that have calories and are the principal energy hotspots for your body. Regardless of where they come from, the calories you eat are either switched over completely to actual energy or put away inside your body as fat. These put away calories will remain in your body as fat except if you go through them. You can do this by cutting the number of calories you that take in so your body should draw on saves for energy. Or on the other hand you can add more exercise with the goal that you burn more calories. Your weight is a difficult exercise, yet the condition is basic. Assuming that you eat a larger number of calories than you burn, you put on weight.

Furthermore, on the off chance that you eat fewer calories and perform more work, you get more fit.

Previously, research found around 3,500 calories of energy rose to around 1 pound (0.45 kilogram) of fat. So specialists thought consuming or cutting 500 calories daily prompted losing 1 pound seven days. In any case, this isn't valid for everybody.

Generally, in the event that you cut around 500 calories per day from your standard eating routine, you might lose about ½ to 1 pound a week. In any case, this can fluctuate contingent upon your body, how much weight you need to lose, and your orientation and action level.

It sounds straightforward. Be that as it may, it's more troublesome in light of the fact that when you get thinner, you as a rule lose a blend of fat, lean tissue and water. Likewise, due to changes that happen in the body as a reason for weight reduction, you might have to diminish calories more to continue to get thinner. Slicing calories needs to incorporate change; however it doesn't need to be hard. These progressions can hugely affect the quantity of calories you take in:

- Skirting unhealthy, low-sustenance things
- Trading fatty food sources for lower calorie decisions
- Portion reduction

Skirting a couple of fatty things could be a decent spot to begin while cutting calories. For instance, you could skirt your morning latte, soft drink at lunch, or that night bowl of frozen yogurt. Ponder what you eat and drink every day and find things you could remove. Assuming you believe that skirting your treat will leave you with a desire, trade it with a low-calorie decision.

Basic trades can have a major effect with regards to cutting calories. For instance, you can save 60 calories a glass by drinking without fat milk rather than entire milk. Rather than having a second cut of pizza, go after some new organic product. Or then again nibble on air-popped popcorn rather than chips. Eat more products of the soil, which have numerous supplements and are high in fiber. Also, they'll top you off more than high-fat decisions.

Portion Control

The size of your food portion influences the number of calories that you're getting. Two times the quantity of food can once in a while mean two times the quantity of calories. Yet, a few food sources with fewer calories, like many products of the soil, can be eaten in bigger bits.

It's generally expected to figure that you eat short of what you really do, for example, assuming you're feasting out. Focusing on your bits is an effective method for controlling calories.

Attempt these tips to control segment sizes and cut calories:

Begin little: Toward the beginning of a dinner, take somewhat less than your thought process you'll eat. Assuming you're as yet eager, eat more vegetables or natural product.

Eat from plates, not bundles: Eating right from a holder provides you with no feeling of the amount you're eating. Seeing food on a plate or in a bowl keeps you mindful of the amount you're eating. Contemplate utilizing a more modest plate or bowl.

Check food marks: Make certain to check the Sustenance Realities board for the serving size and number of calories per serving. You might find that the little sack of chips you have with lunch consistently, for instance, is two servings, not one. This implies it's two times the calories you thought.

Utilize a calorie counter: Look at trustworthy assets that deal with instruments to count calories, like sites or cell phone applications.

Supplanting unhealthy food sources with lower calorie decisions and cutting your piece sizes can assist you with cutting calories and further develop weight control. For an effective and enduring weight, you likewise need to expand your exercise. Consolidating standard action and good dieting will aid you in achieving and keeping a solid weight.

Chapter 7

Metabolism and how it affects Weight Loss

You've likely heard individuals pin their weight on an inability to burn calories, yet what's the significance here? Is metabolism actually the guilty party? Also, assuming this is the case, is it conceivable to speed up your metabolism to burn more calories?

The facts confirm that metabolism is connected to weight. However, in opposition to normal conviction, a sub-optimal ability to burn calories is seldom the reason for excessive weight gain.

In spite of the fact that your metabolism impacts your body's essential energy needs, the amount you eat and drink along with how much exercise you get, are the things that eventually decide your weight.

Metabolism is the cycle by which your body changes over what you eat and drink into energy. During this perplexing system, calories in food and drinks are joined with oxygen to deliver the energy your body needs to work.

In any event, when you're very still, your body needs energy for all its "covered up" capabilities, for example, breathing, coursing blood, changing chemical levels, and developing and fixing cells. The quantity of calories your body uses to complete these essential capabilities is known as your basal metabolic rate — what you could call metabolism.

A few elements decide your individual basal metabolism, including:

Your body size and arrangement: Individuals who are bigger or have more muscle burn more calories, even very still.

Your sex: Men generally have less muscle versus fat and more muscle than do ladies of a similar age and weight, and that implies men burn more calories.

Your age: As you age, muscle will in general diminish and fat records for a greater amount of your weight, dialing back calorie consuming.

Energy needs for your body's fundamental capabilities stay genuinely steady and aren't handily different.

Notwithstanding your basal metabolic rate, two different variables decide the number of calories your body that burns every day:

Food handling (thermogenesis): Processing, engrossing, moving and putting away the food you eat additionally takes calories. Around 10% of the calories from the carbs and protein you eat are utilized during the assimilation and retention of the food and supplements.

Active work: Exercise — like playing tennis, walking to the store, pursuing the dog and some other development — represent the other calories your body burns every day. Exercise is by a wide margin the most factors of the elements that decide the number of calories you that burn every day.

Researchers call the action you do the entire day that isn't purposeful activity **Non-Exercise Activity Thermogenesis** (NEAT). This movement incorporates walking from one space to another, exercises like planting and in any event, squirming. Perfect records for around 100 to 800 calories utilized day to day.

Metabolism and weight

It very well might be enticing to fault your metabolism for weight gain. But since metabolism is a characteristic nteraction, your body has numerous components that direct it to meet your singular requirements.

Just in uncommon cases do you get exorbitant weight gain from a clinical issue that eases back metabolism, like Cushing's condition or having an underactive thyroid gland (hypothyroidism).

Sadly, weight gain is a muddled cycle. It's probable a mix of hereditary cosmetics, hormonal controls, diet organization and the effect of climate on your way of life, ncluding rest, exercise and stress.

These elements bring about lopsidedness in the energy condition. You put on weight when you eat a larger number of calories than you burn— or burn fewer calories than you eat.

While the facts confirm that certain individuals appear to be ready to get in shape more rapidly and more effectively than others, everybody sheds pounds when they burn a bigger number of calories than they eat. To get thinner, you really want to make an energy shortage by eating fewer calories and expanding the quantity of calories you burn via exercise.

While you don't have a lot of command over the speed of your basal metabolism, you have some control over the number of calories that you burn and the degree of exercise you partake in. The more dynamic you are; the more calories you burn. As a matter of fact, certain individuals who are said to have a quick metabolism are most likely more dynamic — and perhaps squirm more — than others.

Try not to seek dietary enhancements for help in burning calories or weight reduction. Items that case to accelerate your metabolism are much of the time more promotion than help and some might cause bothersome or even risky secondary effects.

Dietary enhancement makers aren't needed by the U.S. Food and Medication Organization to demonstrate that their items are protected or compelling, so view these items with alert. Continuously let your PCPs in on about any enhancements you take.

There's no simple method for getting in shape. The establishment for weight reduction keeps on being founded on physical activity and diet. Take in fewer calories than you burn, and you get in shape.

The Dietary Rules for Americans prescribes slicing calories by 500 to 700 calories every day to lose 1 to 1.5 pounds (0.5 to 0.7 kilograms) seven days. On the off chance that you can add consume exercise to your day, you'll achieve your weight reduction objectives much quicker.

www.ingramcontent.com/pod-product-compliance
Lightning Source LLC
LaVergne TN
LVHW050338160826
845677LV00014B/3672

9798353042563